Michael Winicott

EMPOWER YOUR

BRAIN

Work out your brain to increase intelligence and memory

Published by UNITEXTO
www.unitexto.com info@unitexto.com

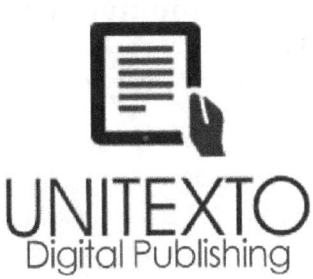

UNITEXTO
Digital Publishing

Table of Contents

1. Introduction

Intelligence is one of the things all of us have definitely thought of numerous times, but do we really have a clear idea about what it is? Have you asked yourself what makes someone very smart and what it takes to qualify as such? Did you find a complex and satisfactory answer? How would you define intelligence? Is being smart a matter of innate endowment or is intelligence mere potential that you can activate and use constructively or alternatively dissipate?

In this book I will share the best methods for maintaining not only an active mind, but a brain whose powers tap into resources that may be latent. I will introduce you to the vital means of increasing your intelligence and learning new things the best way possible. The book will focus on activities designed to stimulate your mind and directly make you smarter such as seeking new experiences and facts, stimulating your creativity, enhancing abstract reasoning skills, playing strategy games, solving puzzles, and other practices that you may not have even suspected to be among the secrets of smart people.

2. What Is Intelligence and What Do Smart People Have?

2.1. Common Preconceptions about Intelligence

Intelligence is usually associated with the ability to think abstractly, find solutions and strategies, understand and process complex ideas, design elaborate plans that make things work, think logically and make sense of things around us, and not least easily assimilate new information. However it is crystal clear that intelligence is far more than being book smart and having learned facts about various things and phenomena.

For example, it is also the ability to learn from experience and adjust our tools to meet new demands. Emphasizing this quality, Stephen Hawking said that intelligence is the ability to adapt to change. Of course being smart is more than that, but we should be aware of the complexity of intelligence and not misunderstand it by focusing on one or two aspects only.

We're commonly tempted to think intelligence is best defined as problem-solving ability, especially when we relate it to what is usually measured through IQ tests. Nevertheless these are fairly standardized and the very concept of IQ is challenged by other notions such as emotional intelligence or social intelligence. You have probably already heard of Howard Gardner's theory about multiple types of intelligence which categorizes people's smarts according to different criteria (e.g. intrapersonal, bodily-kinaesthetic, or spatial) instead of one single standard of measurement implied by IQ.

Apart from challenging the notion of a unique intelligence as well as the frame for assessing it, such theories also question the idea that intelligence is a "given", a gift from birth that people have to live with and cannot influence by sheer force of will and training.

With such notions, how can we still take intelligence for inborn skill only? Have you ever known anyone who showed extraordinary gift from an incredibly early age and maintained that ability in the same form all their life? Have you ever met anyone so closed-minded and rigidly set in their unsatisfactory ways, that they couldn't learn new things and challenge their mental capacities? Experience showed me the opposite is actually true: we can increase our intelligence. If you start from the premise that you cannot shape your own mental capacities, you have already lost the battle. Why so? Because our intelligence is a fluid and flexible gift and its potential is almost unlimited. We shouldn't only measure intelligence through the vastness of our knowledge. Some people know a lot, but have little use for what they know and have memorized.

2.2 Can You Be Truly Intelligent If You Don't Want to Become Even Smarter?

Plutarch said that intelligence is not a vessel to be filled, but a fire to be kindled. We are the ones who have to maintain that fire and make sure it lightens the rest of our lives, since stagnation or the belief that our intelligence has strict and insuperable limits equals a form of mental death. Of course there are callings and types of activities that we can do better than others; however at the same time there are myriad ways we can become smarter than we already are. All we have to do is train our brains the right way! How can we do that?

The bottom line is that being satisfied with what we already have or can do and yielding to a state of passivity is the best way of killing our potential of gaining more mental skills. There's invaluable truth to be extracted from the clever words of someone like Einstein: "One should not pursue goals that are easily achieved. One must develop an instinct for what one can just barely achieve through one's greatest efforts."

This brings us to one of the deepest golden rules about intelligence: being exceptionally smart may actually mean knowing how you can become even smarter than you already are. Intelligence is the awareness that you have limits to challenge and overcome, not to be taken down by. People who are unanimously considered to be smart are extremely attuned to the secrets of maintaining their intelligence in an active state and of increasing their mental capacity. They know what it takes to develop extra skills and they practice their truth almost like a creed, because they value intelligence a lot. It is this kind of secrets and immensely valuable knowledge that you'll tap into through this book. You'll discover that it is not actually exhaustingly difficult to increase your intelligence. You only have to know the best methods and start in full awareness of how malleable our mental abilities are.

3. Top Methods for Training Your Brain and Being Smarter

Now that you are reassured that you can grow smarter than you are, let's see what you can do to improve your mental skills. I must mention that by intelligence I don't necessarily mean IQ, the IQ we all know which is usually evaluated in standardized tests. When I talk about intelligence, I refer to all aspects of such a quality. However let's not ignore the fact that sharpening your "brain power" will also result in your getting better results in such tests, in case you need them for job applications or other endeavours.

3.1. Seeking New Experiences

The first step towards getting smarter is committing not to your habits and your known ways, but to seeking what's new and not yet trodden. Does it sound paradoxical? Of course habitual practice can make perfect and we all pride ourselves on our expertise that took years to acquire. However we must go beyond that if we want to activate more of our mental potential. We shouldn't grow too satisfied with what we already know. Let's say the best way to avoid stagnation or, better yet, "fossilization" is to be extremely open to learning novel things and approaching what we already know from new perspectives, with fresher eyes and more modern tools.

Does it sound difficult and even exhausting? Maybe you are thinking there are people who have invested much of their lives in training so as to get to "blindly" know their way in a field and master a skill easily, as a pro. Wouldn't focusing on something new prove to be detrimental to what they already specialise in? The answer is no. Learning new things and staying open to "the unknown" only helps you develop more dexterity in handling what you already know and it guarantees your brain stays in a state of openness and adaptability to new methods and info. Only this way can you train your mental powers, not by growing complacent and totally convinced that there's no place for getting better and finding out more.

You have probably heard about The Big Five theory. Did you know that people who score high in openness have much more chances of increasing their intelligence? This personality trait that appears independent and seems to relate to character (or charisma) rather than to intelligence is actually one of the secret weapons of smart people. How come? It's simple: openness is tightly connected with the thirst for new activities and new information. It enables you to absorb new facts and acquire new skills on a constant basis. Seek new experiences, even if at first they may seem too strange or irrelevant for your job or your lifestyle! Getting in contact with novel ideas, new places, innovative ventures etc. will result in an increased ability to retain and process information on the long run.

Did you know that seeking novel experiences triggers dopamine? In its turn, this contributes to the creation of new neurons in your brain. Your brain is always ready to learn new things, since this complex series of processes is already part of the way it functions. It's up to you to use it to its best potential and not let it ossify. Neurogenesis goes hand in hand with the so-called synaptic plasticity. Does it sound too abstract and scientific? Well, it is not. This notion stands for our brain's ability to make new connections and learn new things.

3.2. Stimulating Your Creative Thinking

Creativity is the key to intelligence. People who are considered geniuses started from exploring the unsuspected and seemingly unattainable. Creativity can be losing yourself in forms of brainstorming, even though at first sight they don't necessarily look like they will lead somewhere specific. Creativity boils down encouraging divergent thinking. Being creative doesn't only mean engaging in arts or writing poetry.

There are myriad ways of stimulating your brain to think outside the box. While convergent thinking implies following a series of well-known logical steps in order to reach one single solution, the optimal one for a situation or problem, divergent thinking doesn't limit you to one direction only, but urges you to explore multiple paths and thus discover facets of truth that you may have not known before. This is a perfect way of enhancing your mental prowess, since you're not sticking to an already known route in your thought processes; on the contrary, you are offering your mind the right contexts to act spontaneously, in a free-flowing and flexible way. Thus it can find creative solutions on its own, not by attempting to respond to already familiar standards.

3.3. Setting Challenging Goals

Nobody feels stimulated by goals that are too easy to achieve. This principle is valid for the way your brain works, too. Your intelligence increases as you expose yourself to more difficult problems and strive to solve them. Beyond the purely pragmatic interest that governs our lives, our brain demands constant challenge or else its powers weaken. Why should we not tap into its latent potential?

Challenge stops when we notice we master something and we don't have to make extra efforts to get better results. Some of you are probably experts at chess or less complicated things such as video games. Have you ever felt there's a threshold to your pleasure of winning? Don't you get bored when you don't have a worthy opponent, one who makes you question your own skills and indirectly urges you to learn new things, even their own tricks?

The key to providing your brain the constant challenge that it needs on a deeper level is to put aside activities that you grow very good at. Did you learn a new game? Great. If you master it, consider it enough for a good while and move on to your next challenge. Obviously I'm not saying you should take up a totally new profession when you're 50. If you're a language teacher, getting into construction work only to experience a feeling of hardship is ludicrous. Take up a related hobby, learn to play an instrument apart from your "serious" work, start acquiring knowledge in a new language, or enroll in some new course that can help you stay active and mentally stimulated!

Additionally you can surround yourself by highly trained and proficient colleagues, even if this may make you feel a bit doubtful, insecure, and even embarrassed at first. You'll feel competitive and challenged and after enough time you'll be able to be proud of yourself for learning something new and testing your limits. In the end you'll feel newly satisfied with having grown a bit smarter instead of dull and plain.

There is scientific proof that your brain experiences higher levels of energy after weeks of engaging in a new and challenging activity. This leads to more neural connections as you become an expert in something you didn't master before. There's an increased amount of glucose in your brain when you make efforts to learn new things and there's a growth in cortical thickness which stops once you don't have to strain in order to overcome some degree of difficulty.

For this reason it's best to initiate some new activity and learn "the hard way" on a regular basis. Think at long-term effects as well: as you grow older, you'll combat the imminent weakening of your mental powers if you train your mind to get accustomed to challenging things early on. The truth is modern technology often makes our lives easier and more comfortable, but it also teaches us to try to save time and do things at high speed for the sake of efficiency instead of putting our own skills to new tests.

Enjoy its irreplaceable benefits, but don't let technological developments prevent you from growing smarter! Your computer should not do everything for you and your GPS may actually steal the challenge from yourself. Have you thought about that? If you haven't, it's about time you did.

3.4. The Importance of Networking

As an all-encompassing way of keeping your brain up-to-date and regularly challenged through fresh information and facts, networking is invaluable. Connecting with other people makes you stay tuned to new perspectives and info in one of the most natural ways. You will have an enjoyable way of letting fresh facts flow into your life, as you won't have many risks of becoming narrow-minded and wrapped in your own thinking patterns.

This is especially recommendable for those of you who have introverted tendencies and are prone to retreat in their own minds rather than be more expansive and dive in new experiences (and even social relationships) as a second nature. If you know you tend to rely mostly on your own assessment tools and "inner forum", how about becoming more open to others and networking more for a change? Surprising as it may seem, this will not only lead to improved social life, but will ensure your brain stays "tuned". You won't have time to get to lazy when you constantly have to pay attention to what others do, say, or to how they challenge your usual understanding or skills.

3.5. Using Strategy Games and Crosswords

Playing strategy games, video games, or crosswords are all quite good and tested ways of amplifying your brain powers. If you play them together with other people and you enter a quasi-serious competition, it's even better, because you will thus stimulate not only your intelligence, but also your ambition as well as your adrenaline production.

Don't you like the thrill of the combat, a beneficial sense of struggle? It's all in goodwill and fair play. Play games like Chess, Sudoku, Tetris, Scrabble, or simple puzzles with your friends when you have free time. It's an absolutely prolific and activating practice ...much better than talking latest news (which can actually be quite distressing or disturbing) or making mere chit chat.

Play strategy games and logic games or invent ways of testing your knowledge and your erudition. How about creating your own questionnaires? Ask your friend to come up with a set of questions as well and then combine them to sketch an original and spontaneous tests that will get you both on your toes and make you feel competitive as well as in touch with new facts.

You can use a similar strategy for various kinds of games: who's more erudite? Who can speak English/German/French more fluently and more creatively? Who can solve more sophisticated puzzles? Who can solve more crosswords centered on a given topic? Who can build more captivating and elaborate metaphors for a specific thing?

3.6. How to Debate Productively

Alternatively you can enter debating games with your friends or family. Make sure everyone takes this for what it is: means of becoming smarter, not a form of quarrelling. Take the saying "playing the devil's advocate" to a new level. Do this in a deliberate and goal-oriented way. Choose a topic that is open to controversy and decide on a side you could take and defend through articulate and well-organized arguments.

Pretend you're in a court building a case or at least in a debate club where you have to test your rhetoric and argumentation skills against people who are both your partners and competitors. How much does it matter that you actually hold different beliefs? If you can, do it! Take a side you wouldn't normally support and try to convince someone else of the validity of your arguments. As long as you take this game for what it is, a simple way of practicing logics and argumentations, you have nothing to lose, only more strengths to win. Learn to distinguish valid arguments from sophistic reasoning, fact from falsehood etc.

For instance, you can take a political stand, if you're passionate about politics: gay rights vs. heteronormativity. By learning how to frame your opinions and shape a thesis through what you say you are actually also strengthening your skills in verbally defeating other people whose opinions you disagree with in reality. Turn this game into a valuable learning opportunity that will prove helpful when the need arises.

3.7. How Reading and Writing Can Make Anyone Smarter

Read and write ... as much as you can. If your job doesn't require reading on a regular basis, don't give up on books! Set a golden rule: read at least 3 new books per month in order to see which is better. Growing smarter requires reading voraciously, reading out of passion. This way you get in contact with worlds and standpoints unknown to your beforehand and you can feed off the talent and knowledge of others. Read novels or biographies, if it comes easier to you.

It's not imperative to absorb hard scientific facts. Use audio-learning, if printed text seems too dry and bland. Read on your way back home from work. Read while you're waiting for your kid to finish their classes. Read before you fall asleep.

What about writing? What if you're not talented, how can you write? Well, I'm not talking about writing novels like an expert or embarking on a PhD. You can write your own diary, for instance. Have you ever even tried this? It will automatically stimulate your brain, since you'll have to process your experiences on a different level – not only in an immediate way, but also through your mind's eyes, so to speak. You'll have to find an appropriate voice, a fitting tone, the best language to describe what you have lived and felt and you'll sieve your thoughts through a more complex filter when you have to write with an interlocutor (or reader) in mind, even if that's your alter ego.

You could also write short essays. Just think about something that lingers on your mind one evening: destiny, happiness, urban life, love ...what else? If you try this at least once a week, it will doubtlessly expand your mental horizons and make you smarter. You won't be only *living*, but also *processing* your experiences and even slightly modifying them creatively, playing with their meaning, discovering new meanings. We often miss essential aspects of our lives because we tend to mechanize our daily experiences. It seems easier to simply store what happens and move on to other routines.

3.8. Training Your Abstract Thinking Skills

As a more developed form of the same exercise, try training your capacity for abstract thought. How can this be done? There are a series of ways to go if you want to train your power of conceptualization first and foremost. One of them is getting philosophical. Oh, you don't have to write a treatise! It's enough if you try to give your own definitions of some of the most complex and abstract phenomena in life: divinity, power, humanity, life, truth, faith, ethics etc. Ideally you should write down your answers to all such existential questions and state your personal opinions. No matter how close they are to "encyclopaedia truth", you'll grow smarter and wiser as you try to explain reality around you in its basic forms.

A slightly easier way of stimulating the same aspects of intelligence is playing a game of drawing simple connections and patterns between apparently unrelated objects. Think about 3-4 words that describe objects around you and try to draw associations and link them together by some means: find an idea that you can extract starting from one of them, then look for something related that you can infer from the others. This shouldn't stop at concrete facts about objects; it's your abstract verbal reasoning you're working on! Use deductive reasoning, strip words and their meanings to mere ideas, then connect them all through some abstract thread of meaning despite their being quite disparate vocabulary-wise. Think connotatively, beyond literal meanings! For starters, try out the following set of words and see what you can come up with: glass; baptism; paint; kaleidoscope.

A related practice meant to expand your vocabulary and enrich your descriptive and conceptual abilities comes down to a rather simple game: how well do you know your own language? How familiar are you with words? You have surely encountered many of them, but when asked to actually offer precise and elaborate definitions ...how astute are you? If you are a fan of more spontaneity, browse through a more sophisticated magazine and select a few words you feel you'd have a bit of a harder time explaining, no matter how easily you could use them. Then try to define them in one or two sentences. Do this exercise aloud; it will be more amusing and you'll have better control over your explanations. You'll learn to be more concise, extracting essential meaning of words that are usually part of your passive vocabulary.

3.9. IQ Tests Can Also Stimulate Your Intelligence

Do you like IQ tests? If you do, keep taking various versions! Actually it doesn't have to be all about this standardized measuring, you can also try other tests that focus on your dominant brain hemisphere, your type of intelligence according to Howard Gardner, your Maslow hierarchy of needs, your cognitive profile (visionary, motivational, analytical etc.) ...and the list is potentially unlimited.

Not only will you learn new things about yourself, but also you'll be "forced" to question your usual modes of thinking. You'll be asked things you've probably never wondered about. How could you know this if it has never crossed your mind? Well, that's a great opportunity to expand your mind and discover your genuine opinions on certain things.

Some tests can be really challenging. IQ tests don't only have as an effect a measure of your intelligence quotient. They also help you improve your mental skills. They keep you alert and keep you questioning and they make you face difficult questions and problems which is actually a form of challenge that you shouldn't ignore. You won't actively battle against a team of experts in a given field, but you will try to measure up to a set of questions and demands some specialists use to test your intelligence. Consistent testing and practice certainly lead to significant improvement. All right, maybe you won't get surprisingly higher results the next time you take a tests that focuses on intellectual capacity; you may grow more alert, knowledgeable, and acquainted to difficult issues in the mean time ... until you actually notice an important improvement in your actual scores.

4. Nature or Nurture? Bonus Tips for Enhancing Your Mental Prowess

So far I have focused on targeted activities designed to improve your mental powers. Apart from these things you can practice, there are aspects of lifestyle that can very well contribute to the increasing of intelligence, especially across a broader time span. They include nutrition and other ways of taking care of your physical body that are less obviously, but still quite notably connected to developing your intelligence in a form that you are truly satisfied with.

4.1. A "Smart" Diet

When it comes to diet, there are a few facts that you should know. First and foremost, it's recommendable to consider a higher intake of "mentally stimulating" substances. While I don't deny the beneficial effects of caffeine on the brain, but too much of it can also prove to be harmful, leading to increased anxiety or an artificial sense of energy. For this reason I strongly advise you to consider cocoa and certain powerful herbs such as ginko biloba, ginseng, rosemary, or ginger which can act as real brain stimulants. They increase your concentration powers and improve your memory, apart from having an overall energizing effect on the whole organism, in general.

These can be accompanied or used alternatively with supplements such as Omega-3 fatty acids, Lecithin, or B-complex vitamins. If you don't want to load your body with pills that contain such substances in a rather concentrated form, you can extract them directly from food. Eat a larger quantity of fish, carbohydrates (good ones, namely whole grains), nuts, almonds, cashews, and other seeds, spinach and broccoli (rich in Vitamin C and B-vitamins), avocado, liver and eggs (which contain lecithin and iron in significant quantities), dairy products (a lot of calcium, proteins, vitamin D, and magnesium, all of which are known to stimulate brain activity), and bananas. Plan your diet carefully and include such food in higher quantities in order to ensure a regular intake that can maintain your brain in its best shape.

As you can see, you are invited to nourish and nurture your brain along with your body. Actually in this book I want to remind you of the importance of such a connection. Some things may well be facts you're already familiar with, but you fail to consider on a regular basis. Others might be totally new. For instance, did you know that intermittent fasting has proven to enhance our mental abilities? Ironically it is not only eating certain food that will stimulate your brain, but also refraining from eating. The key is to know how to use both secrets. There's no contradiction here.

There are only different aspects of your brain that are acted upon. Intermittent fasting is known to increase the so-called BDNF (Brain-derived Neurotrophic Factor) which has positive effects on your capacity to memorize new things and to learn new skills. There's a funny phenomenon at play here: while you practice intermittent fasting, your brain cells actually grow. The key is to be informed enough about intermittent fasting and use it the right way.

There is scientific evidence that intermittent fasting benefits the brain, not only the physical body (through its detoxification effects). You can neatly combine your main magic tools in order to get the best results: three days of diet rich in substances listed above can be followed by 1-2 days of fasting. Both will enhance your mental capacity, so this is a great formula that should work perfectly if you make sure you get enough nourishing elements through your food intake in the "normal" days of actively nurturing your organism.

This will prevent you from feeling weak or depleted of energy during the days in which you fast. Alternatively you can fast for half of day only, but I personally recommend the other version, as its effects are more powerful. Meanwhile drink plenty of liquids, ideally herbal teas that also act as stimulants on your brain e.g. rosemary, green tea, ginger, black tea, ginseng, basil etc.

4.2. Your Brain-friendly Lifestyle

I have already stressed the similarity between your brain and your body when it comes to their responses to training. However there's more to this connection and I have to remind you of the old, but definitely wise saying about "mens sana in corpore sano". Your brain needs a lot of energy and this can also be enhanced through psychical exercise. Regular exercise is known to stimulate the birth of new brain cells, namely neurogenesis.

A passive person who doesn't train their body, but leads the life of a couch potato is actually also cutting down a lot of power that their brain could benefit from. Your brain needs to be constantly oxygenated and a great way to do this is to practice sports and engage in numerous outdoor activities. As the blood flow to the brain improves, your mental capacities will become visibly better. You'll feel more energetic in front of tasks that you may find difficult, more ready to take in new information, and your concentration power will be enhanced.

Apart from the actual physical, biological, and neurological processes taking place in your whole body, your overall mood will be much better. Faster and more efficient metabolism equals a much better state of mind. Fitness practices are not only means of losing weight; they help you stay in shape psychologically as well and this will have significant effects on your attitude towards new information and activities.

37

Last, but not least, it is vital for your mental capacity that you get plenty of sleep. If you lead a chaotic (or strongly bohemian) life, you cannot expect to learn many new things, can you? Also if you are a hardcore workaholic who's so task-oriented, that they forget about their own health (either physical, or mental), how long do you think your energy can last? Healthy sleeping patterns play an important role in increasing your intelligence. If you sleep at least 7-8 hours each night, your brain won't experience fatigue and you'll be more apt to assimilate new info and learn new things.

An exhausted mind cannot do much for you, no matter how much you try. Also remember that the best sleep takes place during night hours, not in sheer daylight. If you're a night owl, consider changing your schedule for your own good. Never mind that you may stay up late in order to read or watch lots of documentaries that have great potential to make you smarter. You don't want to undermine your own efforts unwittingly, so make sure you are aware of all the subtle processes that take place in your organism and are very prone to influence your mental capacity.

5. Conclusion

In this book I shared with you the best methods for maintaining not only an active mind, but a brain whose powers tap into resources that may be latent. I outlined vital means of increasing your intelligence and learning new things the best way possible. In my book I tried to encompass all forms of mental improvement, even ones that may be considered to be rather "alternative". I wholeheartedly recommend you to try out all of them and alternate them or simply organize them as they best fit your lifestyle, your age, and your line of work/study.

Apart from the purely informational or strategic sides to increasing your intelligence, there is something more related to attitude and emotional tonus that you should keep in mind: a confident and positive approach to learning new things will always be useful, provided that it doesn't border on conceit or unjustified self-satisfaction. It is the openness that does the trick. It is your ability to assimilate novel skills and facts and your power to overcome difficulty that you should be confident in. Beyond this the Socratic words of wisdom still hold true: if you feel that you only know for sure that you know nothing, you surely have more chances or f setting new challenges for yourself and thus becoming smarter. A strong internal locus of control tops all the other tools that you can use.

Someone who considers to be self responsible for successes as well as failures has more chances of getting smarter. Intelligence also comes down to your ability to learn from mistakes and to see your whole life as a learning experiment in which it's not only the destination that counts, but also the journey. Make the best of it and become as smart as you can get in a conscious and deliberate way!